Preface

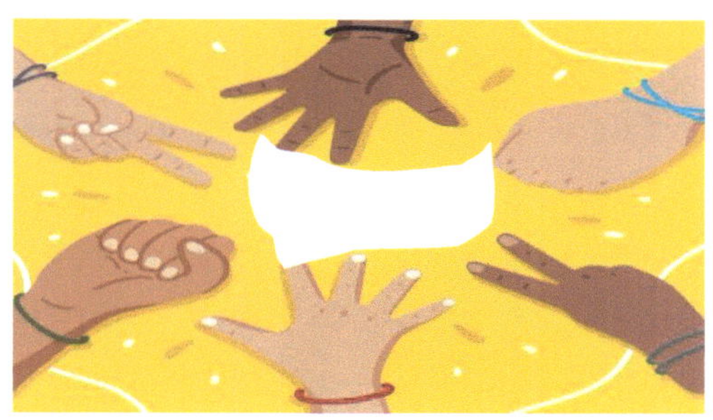

Young's Delight

Volume 4 Series 3

Quarterly Magazine for the youths

Editor: Jane Austin
Tatiana Khabarova,

Jonathan Emmanuel

Published by Brims World

Printed in U.S.A.

Copyright © young's delight

ISBN: 9798873453672

Young's Delight is published by Brims World. In this series the youth are seen as the power source of the world. They are supportive and vibrant to help the world move on. The Youth Day inaugurates seminars and different activities to help them face the challenges of the time they live. We are all here to encourage them to make good things out of whatever comes their way.

Flip through and enjoy!

Jane Austin

Publishing editor

YOUTH AND THE WORLD

Jonathan Emmanuel

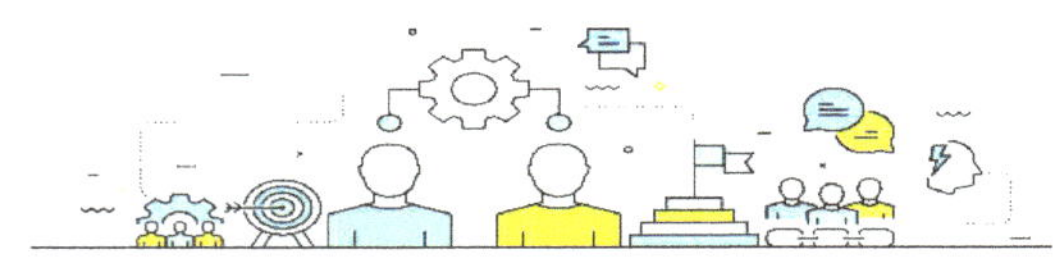

HOW YOUTH AFFECT THE WORLD

Youth can use their energy, creativity, and enthusiasm to create meaningful changes in the world. Youth can play important roles in helping to create more eco-friendly communities by engaging in activities such as recycling, reducing waste, and participating in green initiatives.
This involves efforts to reduce pollution and waste, conserve resources, and maintain an ecological balance.

THE GREATEST NEED OF YOUTH TODAY

Youth feel the need to belong to and be accepted by their peers. Youth are striving for increased freedom from adult controls. There are set reasonable boundaries of behavior. Family members help make decisions on rules and they live within established boundaries. Youth do not like being controlled, therefore, they seek freedom by all means.
The World Programme of Action for Youth, adopted by the General Assembly in 1995, provides a policy framework and practical guidelines for national action and international support to improve the situation of young people around the world. The World Programme of Action for Youth covers fifteen youth priority areas and contains proposals for action in each of these areas.

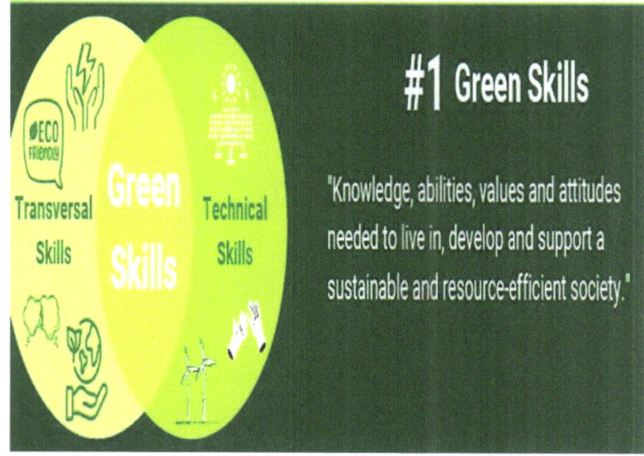

A successful transition towards a greener world will depend on the development of green skills in the population. Green skills are "knowledge, abilities, values and attitudes needed to live in, develop and support a sustainable and resource-efficient society".

These include technical knowledge and skills that enable the effective use of green technologies and processes in occupational settings, as well as transversal skills that draw on a range of knowledge, values and attitudes to facilitate environmentally sustainable decisions in work and in life.

This theme, "Green Skills For Youth: Towards A Sustainable World", International Youth Day 2023.

YOUTH AND THE ENVIRONMENT

WHAT YOUTH NEED TO THRIVE

In teens' words: "Teens thriving means that they are in an environment where they can be completely themselves," and "where their needs, both mental and physical, are heard, understood, and met." Thriving means having "a space of love" and "sharing your ideas with each other and helping people in need.

HOW TO THRIVE

Perspective and approach

Having a positive perspective and an optimistic stance matter to thriving.

Passion and learning

Thriving is also based on development, so embrace your passions and interests.

A bigger picture

Having a large vision is also important.

Relationships

Good relationship matters a lot.

Resilience

Be ready to recover quickly from difficulties or toughness.

Challenges

Be ready to face challenges and prepare to overcome them.

YOUTHS ENLARGEMENT

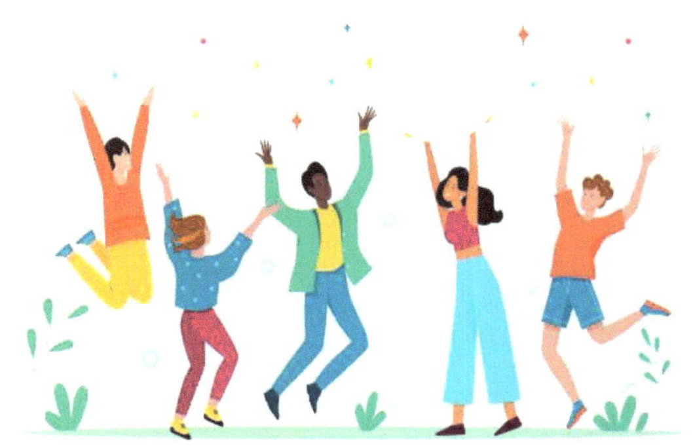

These are the interest of youth today, music, food, fitness, fashion, and sports. They are young consumers' top passions right now.
The following should interest the youth of today:

Learning

Good health

Creativity

Confidence

Future

RECIPE FOR YOUNG HEARTS

SOUPS

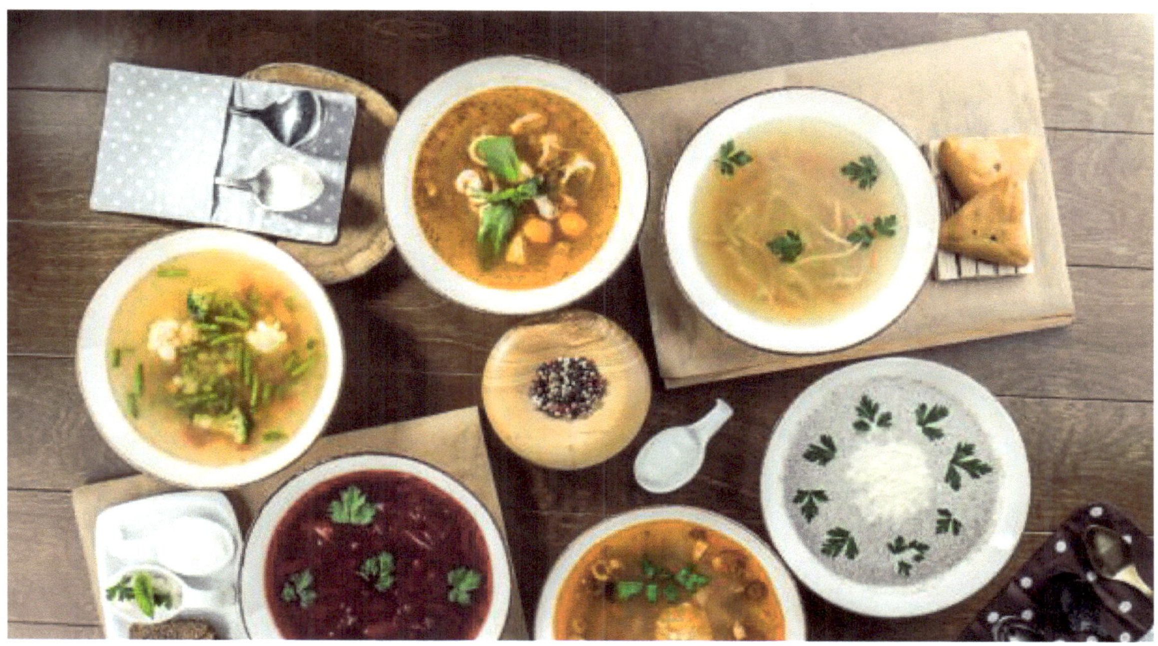

Soups are mostly liquid and they are a great way to stay hydrated and full. They give your immune system a boost. Soups can help you stay off cold and flu. They are a great antidote for times when you are sick too! They are loaded with disease-fighting nutrients.

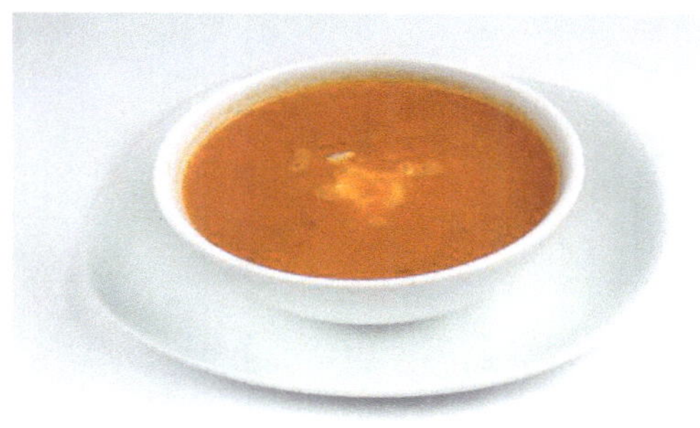

Tomato soup

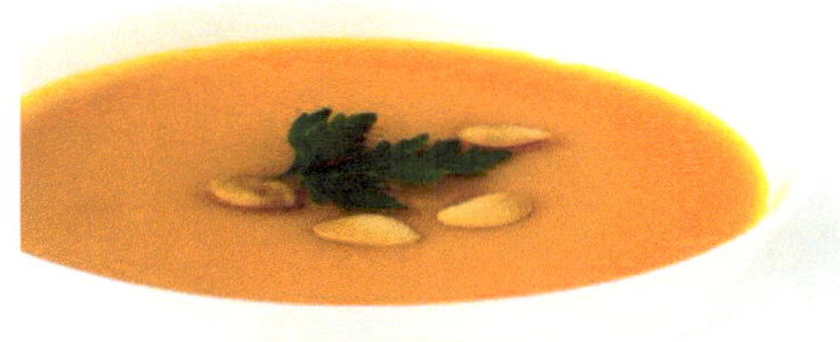

Pumpkin soup

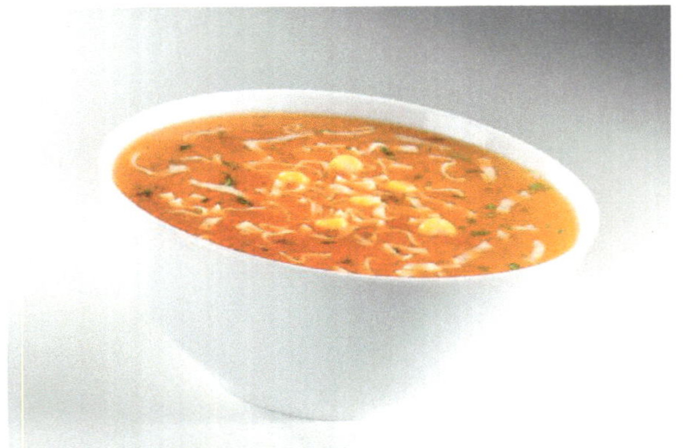

Vegetable cream soup

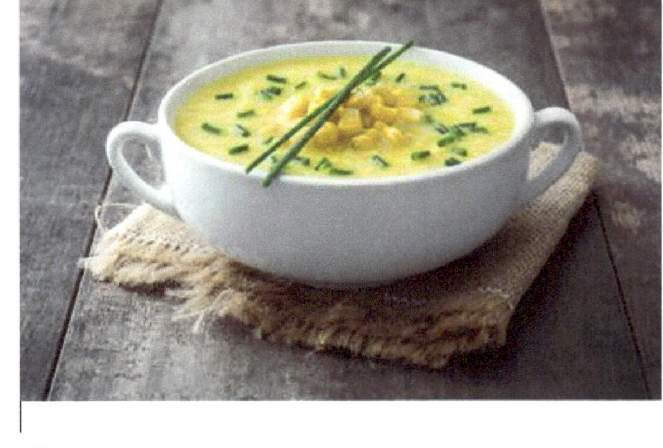

Corn soup

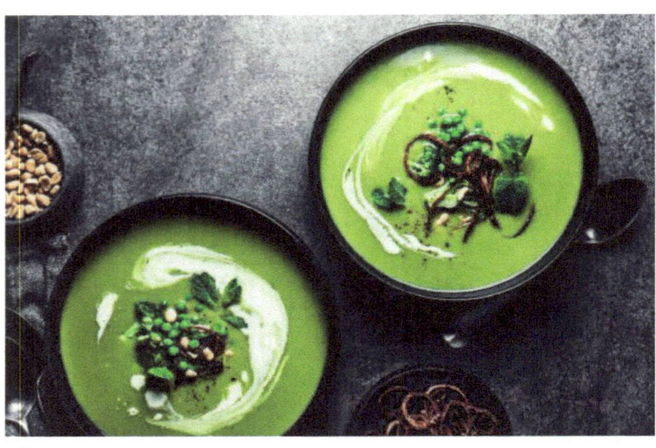

Green peas cream soup

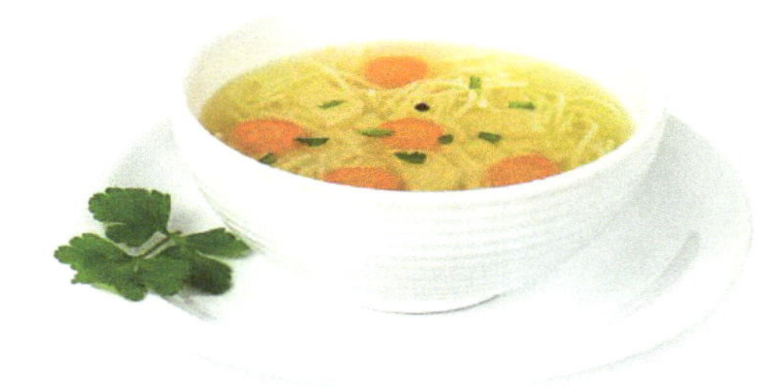

Chicken soup with noodles

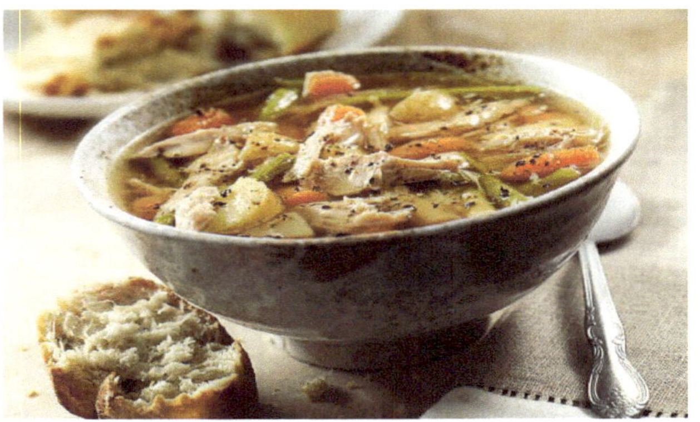

Turkey soup

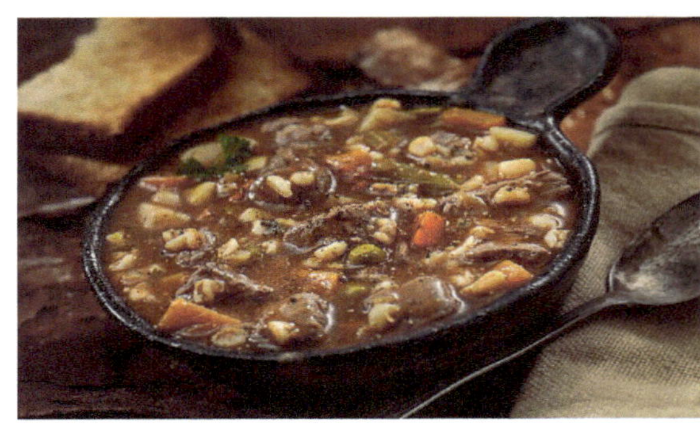

Beef and barley soup

Poetry

MY MOUTH

My mouth contains a tongue

It speaks out words

The words are life and power

 I use it wisely!

My mouth contains some teeth

They are used for biting or eating

The meat I bite and food are eat

How tasty they are!

My mouth is important on my face

I eat and speak with it

I also smile with it

Which makes me lovely!

Social:

YOUTHS WITH DISABILITIES

A YOUTH WITH A DISABILITY

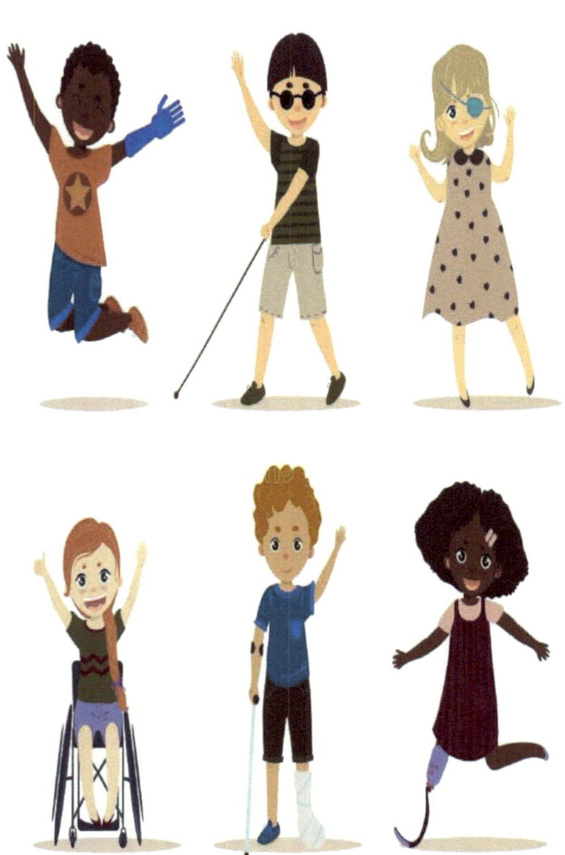

The meaning of a youth with a disability refers to an individual who is handicapped in one or more areas of his or her body.

He or she falls within the range of 14-24 years of age.

Some disabled youths have physical or mental impairment that limits them in major life activities. Some of them have records of such impairments while others like them are regarded as having impairments from birth.

THE STRENGTH OF YOUTHS WITH DISABILITIES

Most people with disabilities have notion for love of learning, honesty, appreciation of beauty and excellence, kindness, and fairness.

POLICY OF EQUAL ACCESS AND OPPORTUNITIES

This action or state of including or of being included within a group is desired by many disabled youth. The practice or policy of providing equal access to opportunities and resources for people who might otherwise be excluded, such as those who have physical or intellectual disabilities and members of other minority groups has become an issue to be resolved. Designing accessible infrastructure and providing equal opportunities for youth with disabilities to participate in all aspects of youth development are equally important in promoting full participation and inclusion of the communities in which they live.

BENEFITS OF EMPOWERING PEOPLE WITH DISABILITY

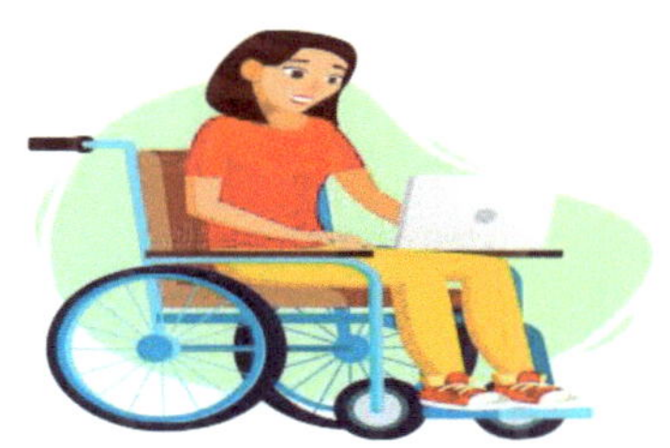

By giving equal opportunities and the corresponding respect, we grow a sense of confidence in the persons with disabilities and cultivate a sense of belonging. This makes for positive growth attitudes, and despite any disability, a person will pursue and work on their goals, thus contributing positively to society.

SIMPLE WAYS TO EMPOWER A PERSON WITH DISABILITY

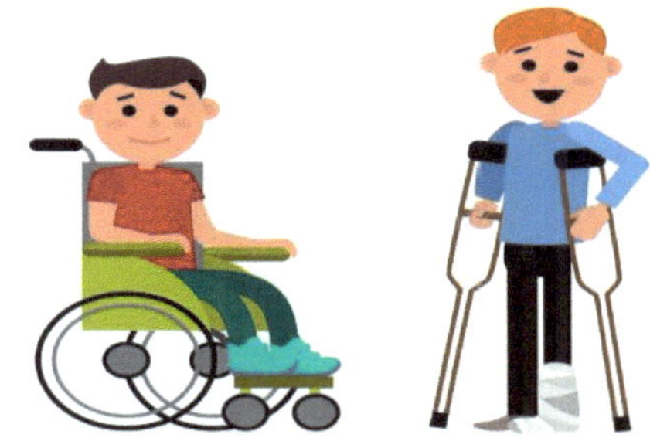

See the person first as disabled
Learn about the person with the disability.
Listen to the person that has the disability.
Encourage decision making to promote independence for people with disabilities.
Promote disability equal access and opportunities.

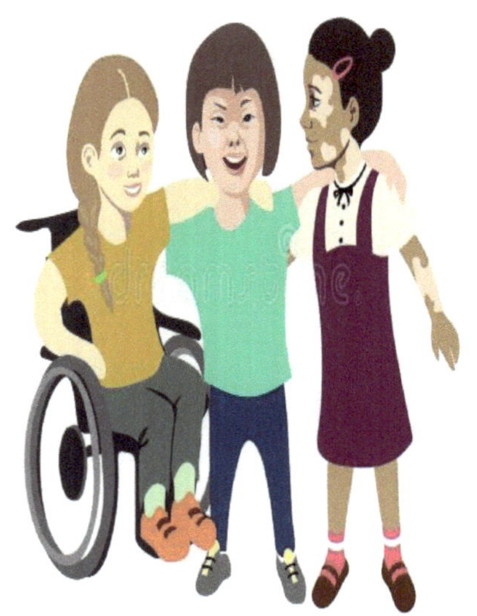

Speak clearly to them to understand what you want to do. And Listen also listen to what they have on mind.

Make them feel confident by assuring them they can.

Respect Personal Space with them. Do not jump on them anyhow to intrude into their privacy.

Make Changes for them by helping them cope with different situations.

Ask Before Offering Help: Do not assume that people with disabilities would always require some assistance in leading their lives and the first step is to treat them as equals. They see themselves as able as yourself.

CAREERS

AGRICULTURE

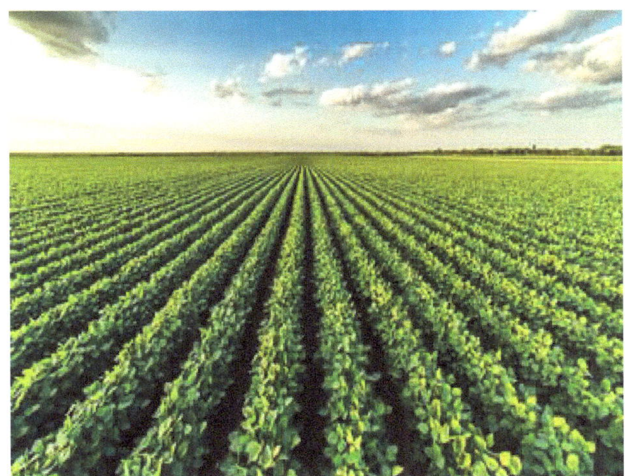

DEFINITION OF AGRICULTURAL PROFESSION

Agriculture careers are professional methods related to farming, cultivation and animal husbandry. These career methods involve everything from growing crops and nurturing the soil to raising livestock like cattle, goats, pigs and chickens, etc.

The most abundant type of agriculture practiced around the world is intensive subsistence agriculture, which is highly dependent on animal power, and is commonly practiced in the humid, tropical regions of the world.

THREE MAJOR AREAS OF AGRICULTURE INDUSTRY

- Agronomy: Agronomy is about the soil, and how the crops will grow in different kinds of soil.
- Agriculture Engineering: Agriculture Engineering is learning about how the different machines work.
- Horticulture: Horticulture is all about the fruits and vegetables and how to grow them.

THERE EXIST FOUR MAIN BRANCHES OF AGRICULTURE, NAMELY

- Livestock production.
- Crop production.
- Agricultural economics.
- Agricultural engineering.

IMPORTANCE OF AGRICULTURE PROFESSION

Agriculture impacts society in many ways, including: supporting livelihoods through food, habitat, and jobs; providing raw materials for food and other products; and building strong economies through trade.

Agriculture provides most of the world's food and fabrics. Cotton, wool, and leather are all agricultural products. Agriculture also provides wood for construction and paper products. These products, as well as the agricultural methods used, may vary from one part of the world to another.

Agriculture is not only used for providing food for human beings and fodder for animals, but it also contributes to the national income of a country.

WHAT A FARMER CAN BE CALLED

Agriculturalist, agriculturist, cultivator, grower, raiser, apiarist, apiculturist, beekeeper.
Someone concerned with the science or art or business of cultivating the soil is a full farmer.

WHAT FARMERS DO

- Planting, fertilizing and harvesting plants.
- Feeding and herding groups of animals.
- Providing special diets and care for animals.
- Collecting food or animal products.
- Performing manual labor.
- Operating farm equipment.
- Selecting and purchasing products such as fertilizer, seeds and equipment.

TOOLS FARMERS USE AND NEED

Quality Tractor

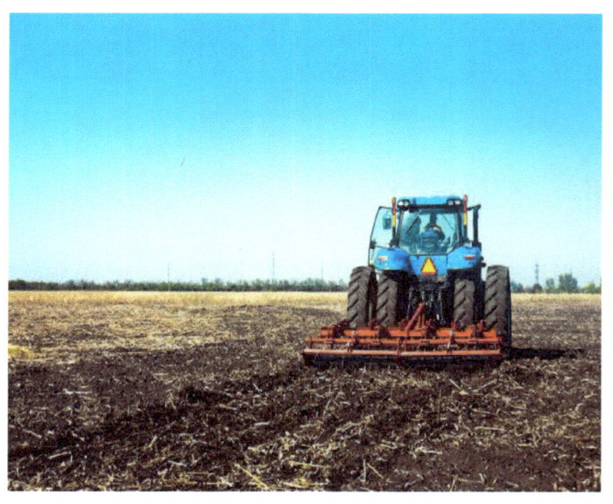

You cannot farm without a tractor because its primary purpose is to pull farming equipment.

Trailers and Wagons

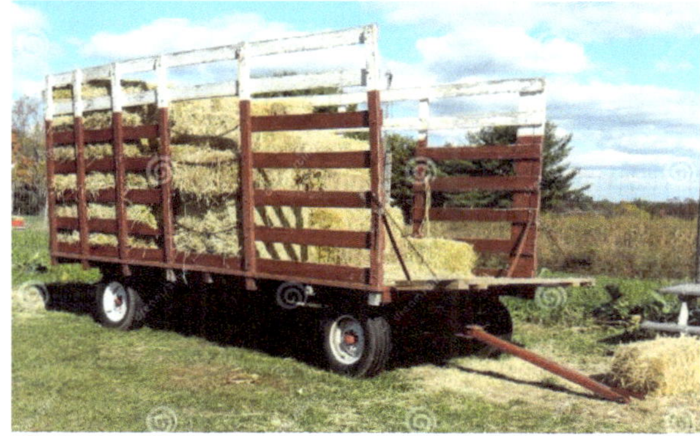

 You can use farm wagons and trailers for numerous purposes, such as:

Harvesters

Comprehensive Irrigation System

Fertilizer Spreaders

Sprayers

Seeders

Rakes

POSITIVE EFFECTS OF AGRICULTURE ON THE ENVIRONMENT

Agricultural systems that work in harmony with nature such as organic, permaculture, or biodynamic farming create diverse natural habitats. For example, open meadow habitats are important for species like waterfowl, amphibians and for pollinators. Some species even increase in number due to agricultural activities.

Agriculture affects the environment in the following ways:

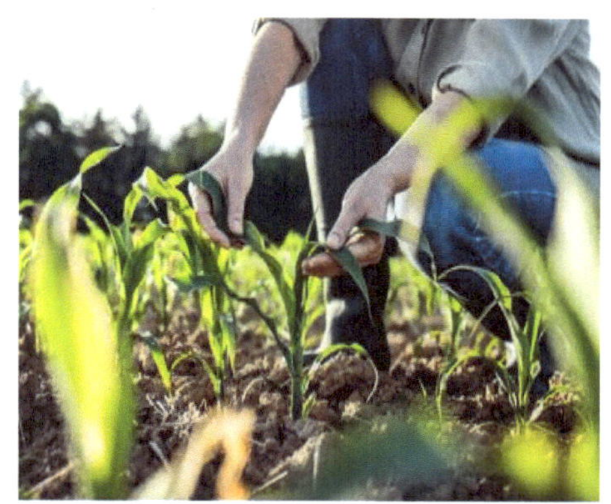

It inspires people.

It preserves ecosystems.

It creates habitats.

It conserves water.

It provides food from limited sources.

 It sets back ecological succession.

It boosts soil fertility.

It sequesters carbon.

retains soil and prevents erosion

YOUTHS AND LEISURE

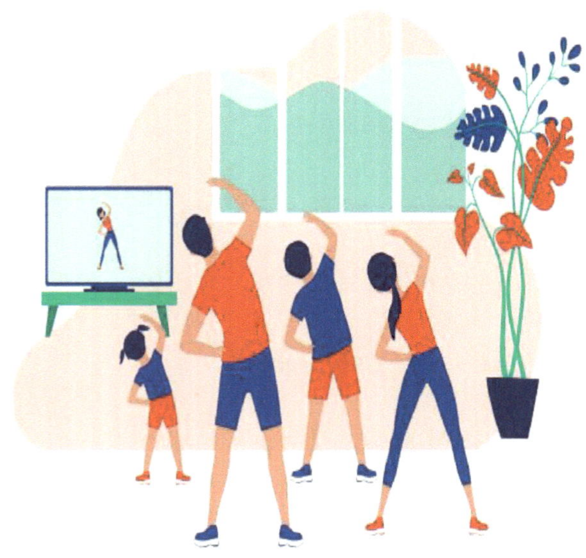

Examples of recreation activities are walking, swimming, meditation, reading, playing games and dancing. Leisure refers to the free time that people can spend away from their everyday responsibilities (e.g. work and domestic tasks) to rest, relax and enjoy l

What are positive leisure activities for youth?

There are several examples of leisure activities. They include surfing, bicycling, traveling, horseback riding, tennis, golfing, skating, walking, swimming, weightlifting, hiking, martial arts, and skiing.

MOST POPULAR LEISURE ACTIVITIES

Most popular hobbies and activities in the world nowadays are:

Video gaming

Outdoor activities

Traveling

 Arts and Crafts

POSITIVE ACTIVITIES

Engaging in hobbies, helping others, re-establishing family routines, and participating in satisfying activities can also improve your mood, make things feel more normal, and restore a sense of control. It may take some time, and it may not feel like fun.

POSITIVE HEALTH OUTCOMES OF LEISURE ACTIVITIES

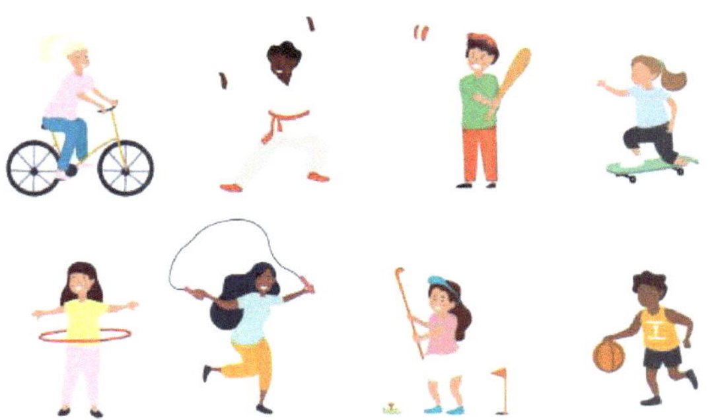

These results in good health when one engages in leisure activities. There are both physical and psychological benefits of leisure time, with reduced levels of stress, anxiety, and depression; improved mood; and higher levels of positive emotion. Engaging in recreational activities can also lower cholesterol levels, blood pressure, and heart rate.

HOW LEISURE HELPS MENTAL HEALTH

Leisure activities are likely to work as a guard against stressful experiences by promoting positive emotions related to self-fulfillment and well-being. Consequently, they work to prevent mental illnesses, such as depression, boredom, etc.

EFFECTS OF LACK OF LEISURE

When we have too little time for leisure we feel stressed and that impacts on our wellbeing. But when we have too much leisure time and do not use it well, we feel unproductive and that also lowers wellbeing.

PRAISES AND SONGS

Jean Forde

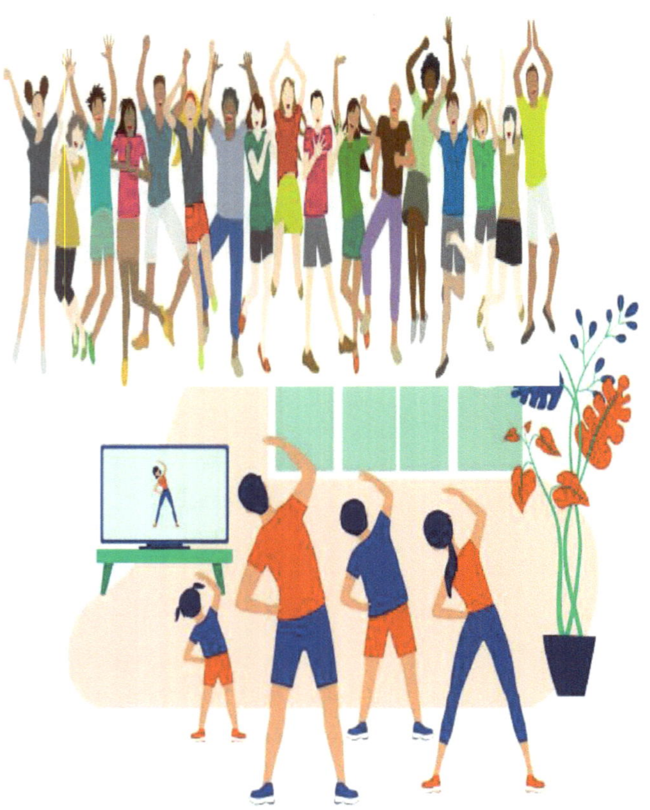

BIBLE VERSES ABOUT PRAISE AND WORSHIP

2 Corinthians 1:3-4. 3 Praise be to the God and Father of our Lord Jesus Christ, the Father of compassion and the God of all comfort.

James 3:10. 10 Out of the same mouth come praise and cursing. Job 1:20-21

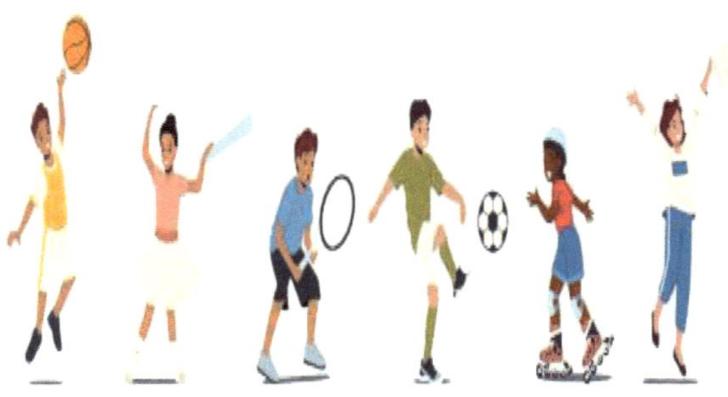

John 4:24

John 4:23

Hebrews 13:15

Isaiah 25:1

Romans 12:1-2.

WHAT THE BIBLE SAY ABOUT PRAISES

Psalm 105:1-2

Oh give thanks to the Lord; call upon his name; make known his deeds among the peoples! Sing to him, sing praises to him; tell of all his wondrous works! Glory in his holy name; let the hearts of those who seek the Lord rejoice.

BIBLE VERSES ABOUT MUSIC

Psalms 95:1. 1 Come, let us sing for joy to the LORD; let us shout aloud to the Rock of our salvation.

Ephesians 5:19. 19 speaking to one another with psalms, hymns, and songs from the Spirit.

Hebrews 2:12. …

Psalms 71:23. …

Exodus 15:1. …

Psalms 105:2. …

Psalms 49:4. …

Psalms 101:1.

WHAT GOD SAY ABOUT SONG

"Sing to him, sing praise to him; tell of all his wonderful acts" (Psalm 105:2). Telling of his wondrous acts not only is a witness to those around us of God's greatness, but it is just as much a blessing to us when we use our voices to speak what God has done for

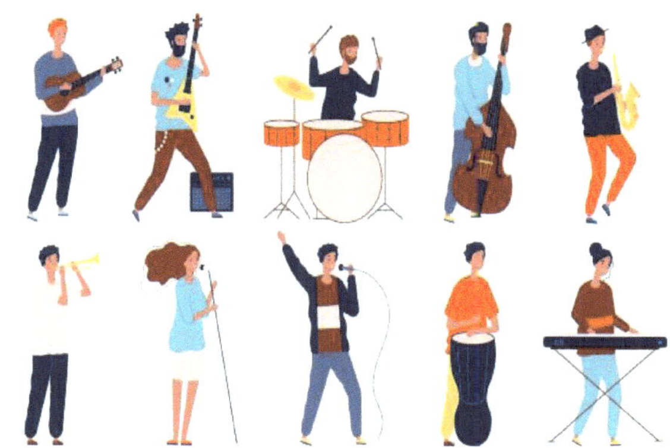

us, reminding us of his goodness.

WHAT THE BIBLE SAY ABOUT SINGING AND MUSIC

Hebrews 2:12 applies Psalm 22:22 to Jesus when it says, "In the midst of the congregation I will sing your praise." And Ephesians 5 tells us that the effect of being "filled with the Spirit" is "addressing one another in psalms and hymns and spiritual songs, singing and making melody to the Lord with your heart"

THE KIND OF MUSIC JESUS WOULD LIKE

Jesus would have appreciated music that brought praise to his Father. He and his disciples often sang Psalms, which are songs of praise.

COLD WEARS

For the youths

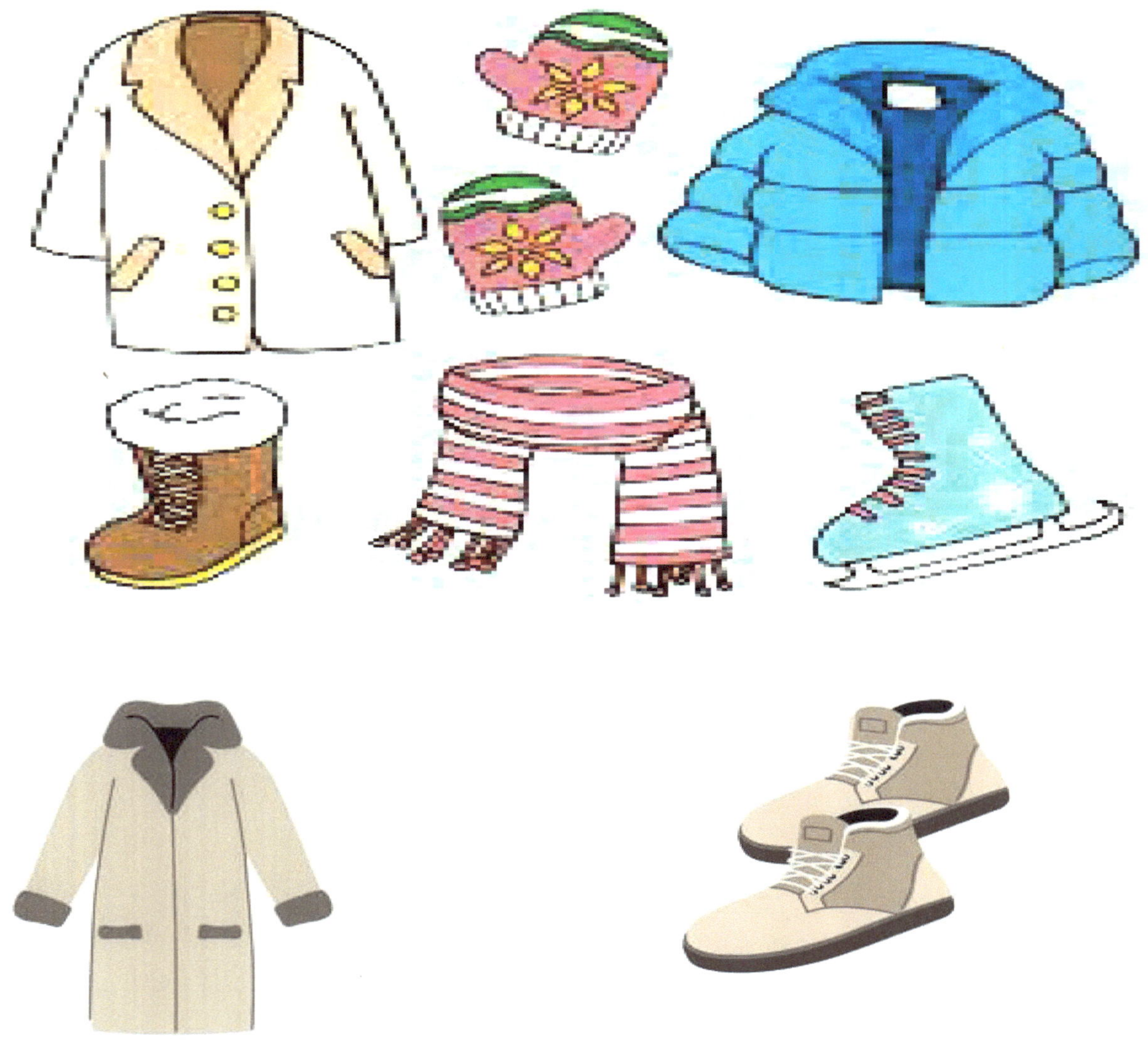

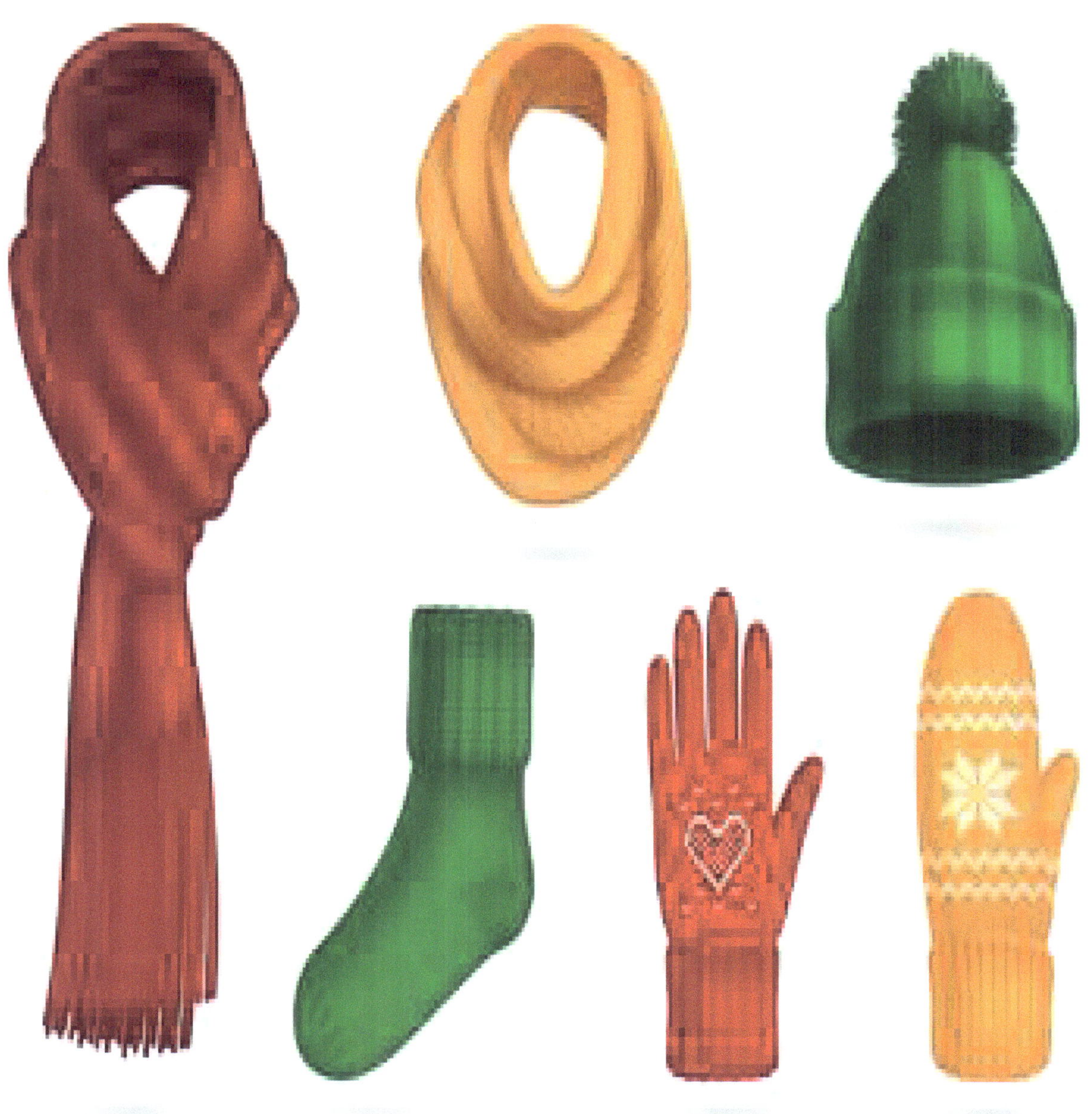

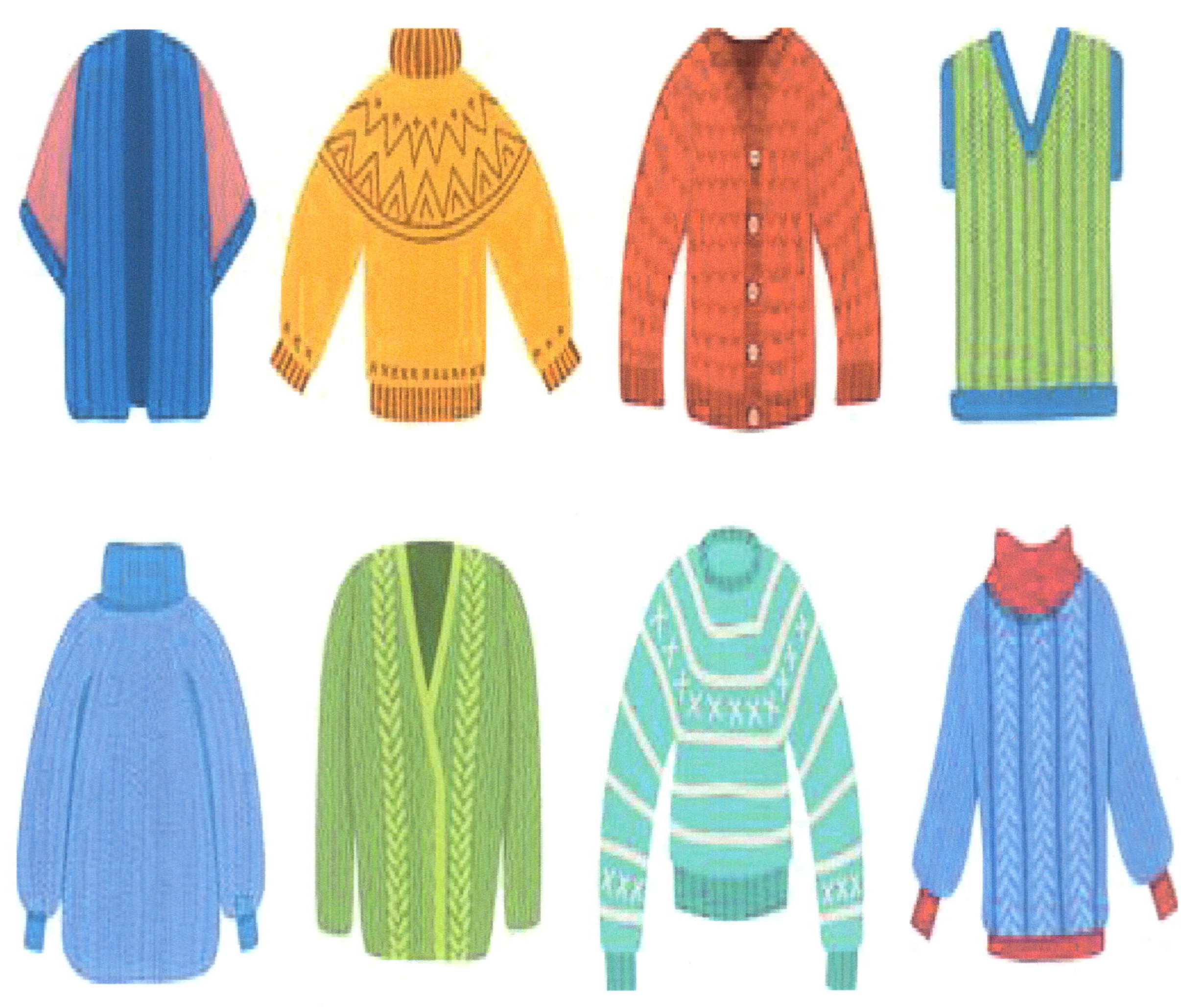

Your Health

Tatiana Khabarova

BREATHING

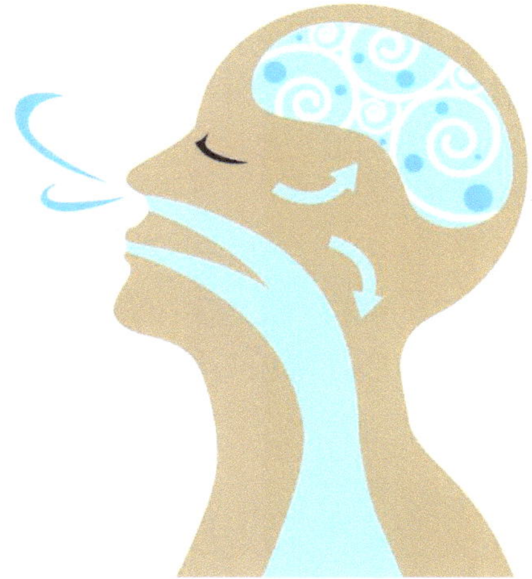

SIMPLE DEEP BREATHING

Deep breathing can help you get closer to reaching your lungs' full capacity. As you slowly inhale, consciously expand your belly with awareness of lowering the diaphragm. Next, expand your ribs, allowing them to float open like wings. Finally, allow the upper chest to expand and lift.

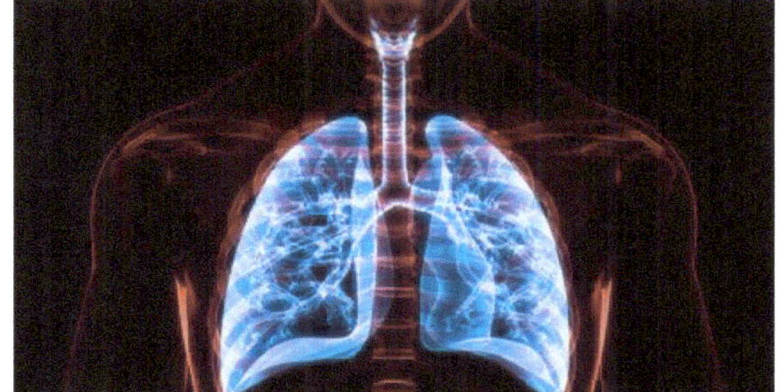

How to know your lungs are healthy. If your breathing is natural, comes easily and not forced, is steady and makes you feel good, or is so regular you do not notice it at all, your lungs are most likely healthy.

HOW TO MAINTAIN EFFECTIVE BREATHING

Regular exercise keeps your lungs functioning well, and a well-balanced diet can help you stay active. Avoid large meals and foods that cause bloating to prevent the abdomen from pushing up and limiting the diaphragm's movement.

THE BEST FOODS FOR LUNG HEALTH

- Beets and beet greens. The vibrantly colored root and greens of the beetroot plant contain compounds that optimize lung function.
- Peppers

- Apples
- Pumpkin
- Turmeric
- Tomato and tomato products
- Blueberries
- Green tea

HERE ARE SOME DRINKS THAT MAY BE BENEFICIAL:

- Green tea. Green tea is rich in antioxidants called catechins, which may have anti-inflammatory and protective effects on lung tissue.
- Turmeric Milk
- Warm water with lemon
- Honey and warm water
- Pineapple juice
- Beetroot juice
- Garlic-infused water

MOST COMMON EARLY WARNING SYMPTOMS:

- Shortness of breath
- Cough that may bring up Sputum, also called mucus or phlegm
- Wheeze or chest tightness
- Fatigue or tiredness

- Reoccurring lung infections like acute bronchitis or pneumonia

HOW TO KNOW LUNGS DEFECTS

The most common symptom is feeling increasingly out of breath. Some people's breathing might get worse much more quickly, over weeks or months. This is particularly true of interstitial lung diseases, such as IPF. For those in the final stages of a lung condition, breathing becomes noticeably worse.

THE BEST POSITION TO SLEEP IN WITH BREATHING PROBLEMS

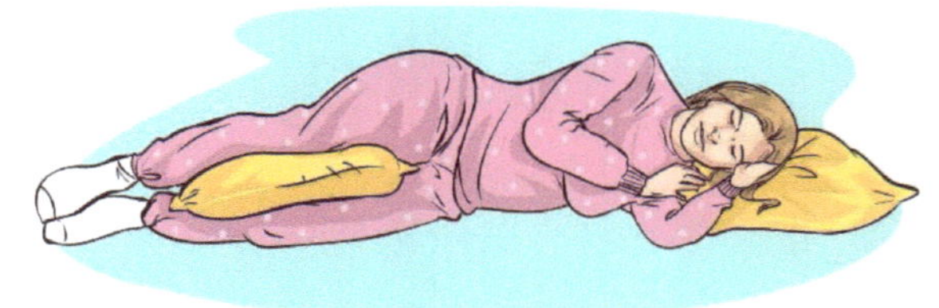

FREEZING!

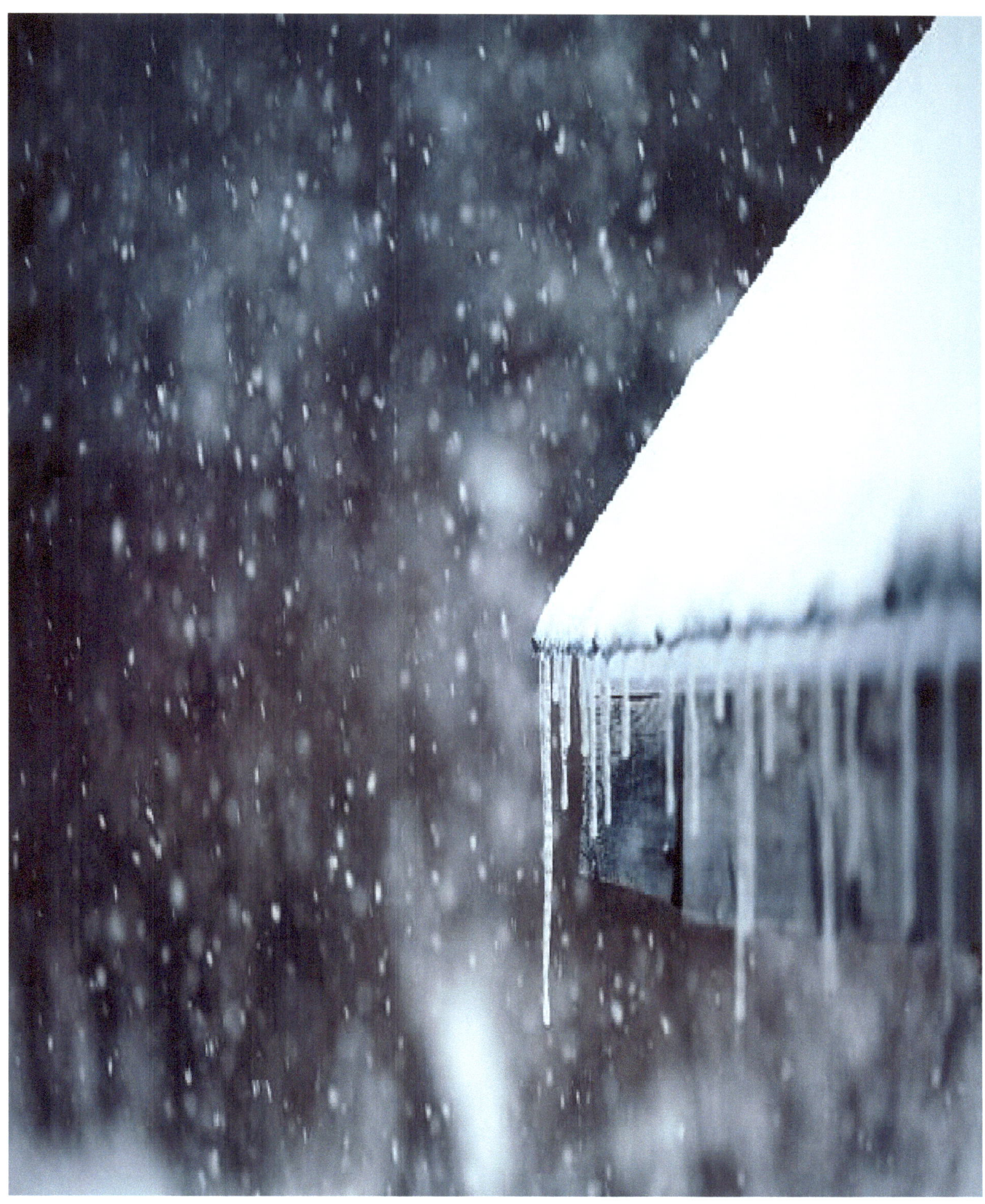

HIGH JUMP

HOW TO PLAY HIGH JUMP GAME

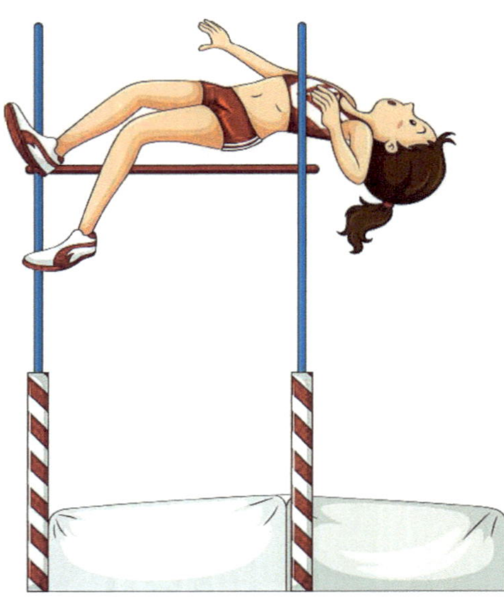

The athlete can run straight or take an angled approach or run fast or slow towards the upright. Once a jumper is near the upright, they airlift vertically using one foot during the take off. The objective is to clear the crossbar placed at a certain height from the ground and land on the crash mat.

THE PHYSICAL QUALITIES TO BE A HIGH JUMPER

The high jump game is a complex track and field event that requires a unique balance. It lies between strength, speed, power, and technique. Athletes must be able to achieve horizontal velocity, convert it to vertical velocity to overcome gravity, and must do all this with special trained technique.

HIGH JUMP RULES

Jumpers must take off from one foot. A jump is considered a failure if the jumper dislodges the bar or touches the ground or any object behind the bar before clearance. Competitors may begin jumping at any height announced by the chief judge, or use a method of their own.

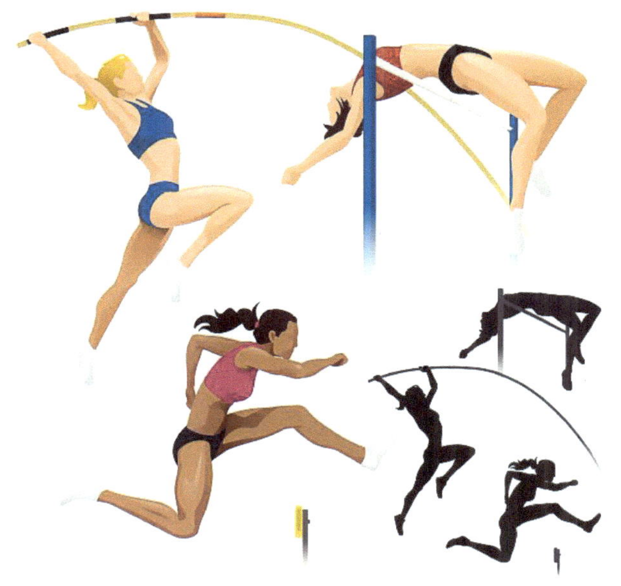

EXERCISE FOR HIGH JUMP TRAINERS

Training to jump high should include movements that build strength,
The following are good exercises;
 Deadlifts
 Squats,
  Tuck-ups
  Box jumps

TERMINOLOGYFOR HIGH JUMP

NH—No Height (vertical jump events such as High Jump and Pole Vault)

A score of 0 in height, where an athlete fails to make a valid jump, in high jump or pole vault, and faults out of competition.

ND—No Distance (throwing and horizontal jump events)

FOOD FOR HIGH JUMP ATHELETES

Protein sources such as meat, fish, eggs, chicken, reduced-fat dairy products, tofu and lentils.

THE THREE BASIC STEPS OF THE HIGH JUMP

The high jump technique is divided into the following phases; approach.
• Take-off,
• bar clearance
• landing.
The take-off is the most important.

PIANO LESSON

Jane Austin

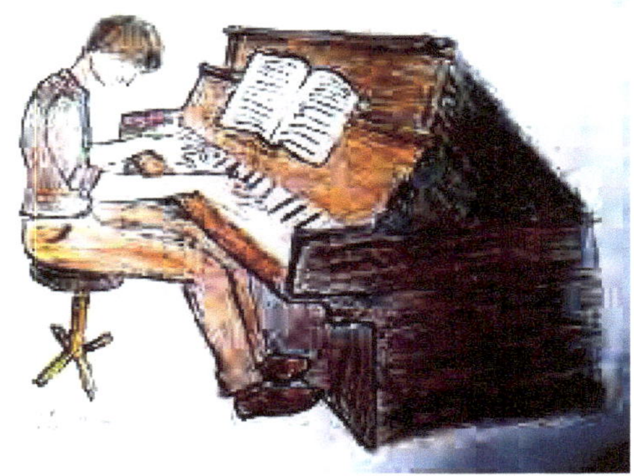

TIPS BEFORE STARTING PIANO LESSONS

1. Make sure you have a reliable instrument.
2. Stay honest with yourself.
3. Learning piano takes practice.
4. Your hands might not move properly right away.
5. Ask Questions.
6. The first step.

THE FIRST THING TO LEARN ON THE PIANO

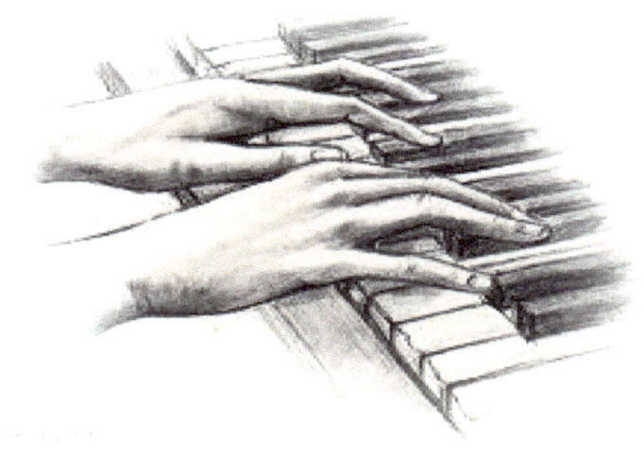

One of the first things you will learn as a new piano player is the layout of the keyboard. You will also learn the musical alphabet and how to form scales and simple chords. Practicing chords and scales can be tedious, but knowing them well will help you to know how to play the keyboard.

PIANO LESSONS FOR A BEGINNER

Reasons for learning piano

Reading music

Playing simple music

Four to twelve lessons

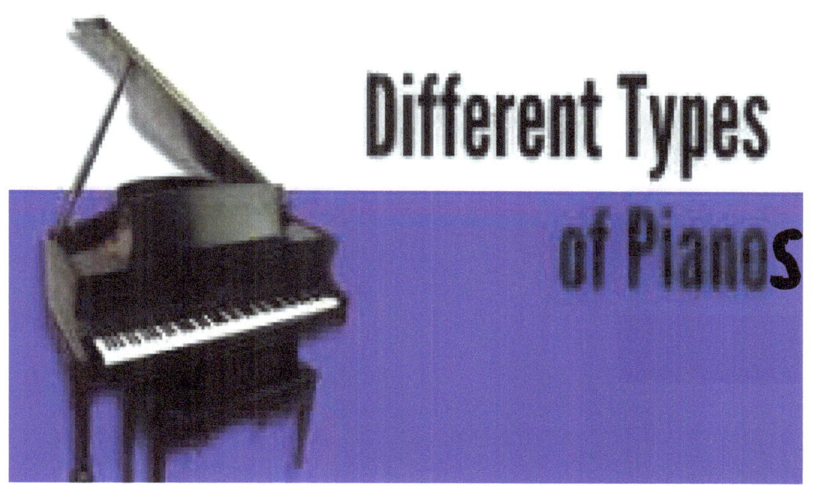

Different Types
of Pianos

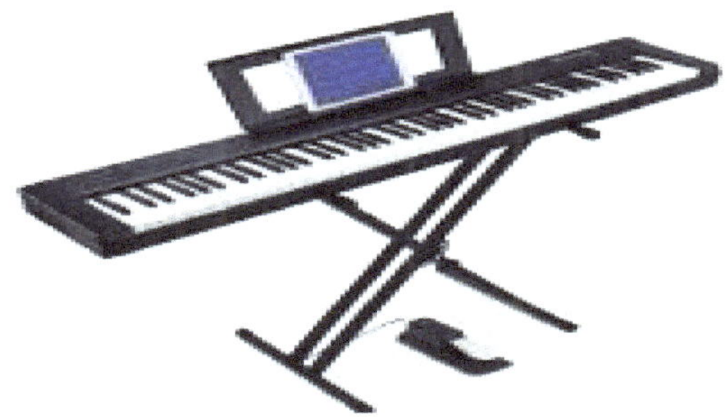

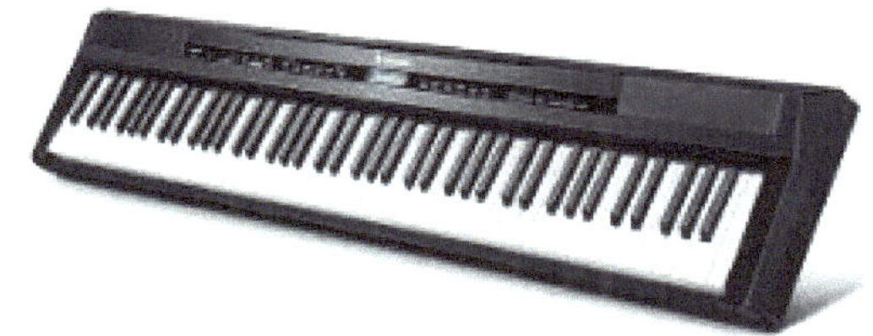

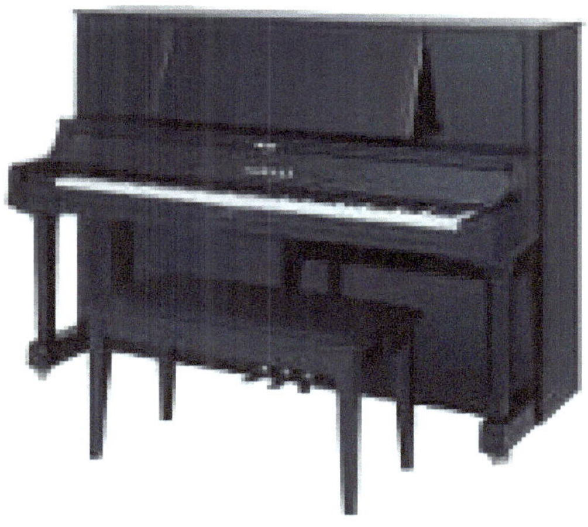

Music cds by Jane Landey

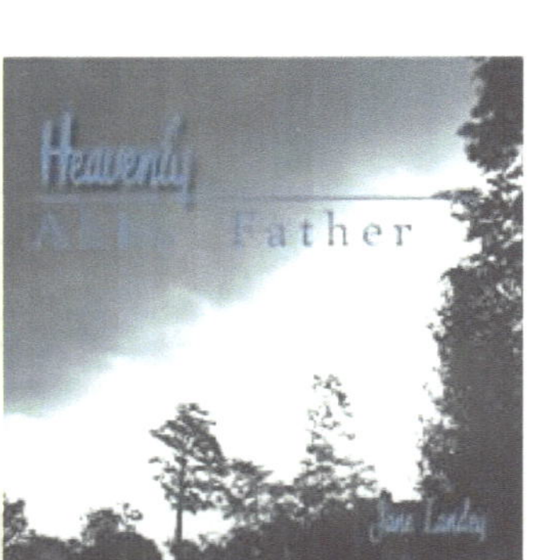

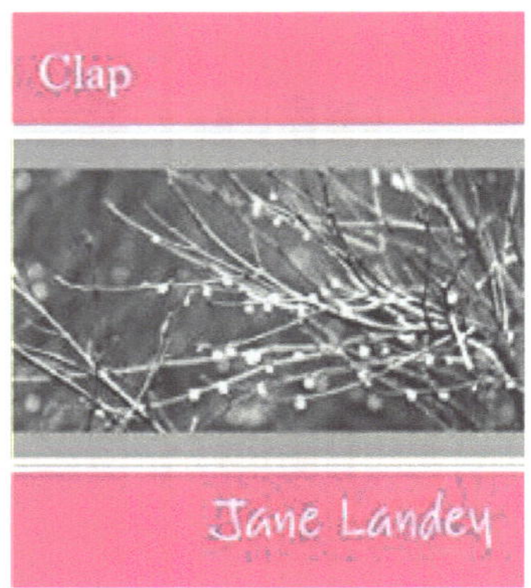

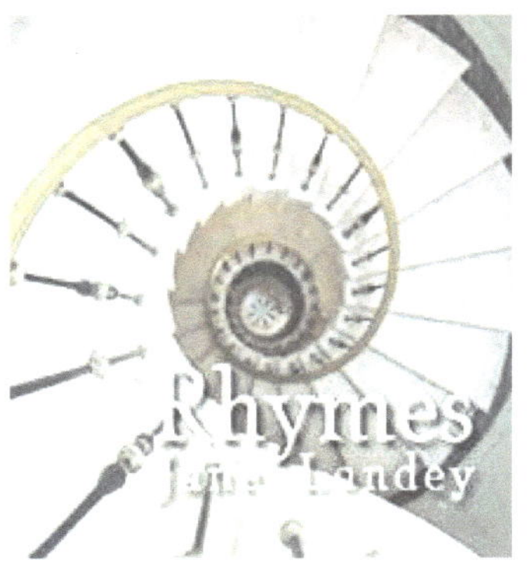

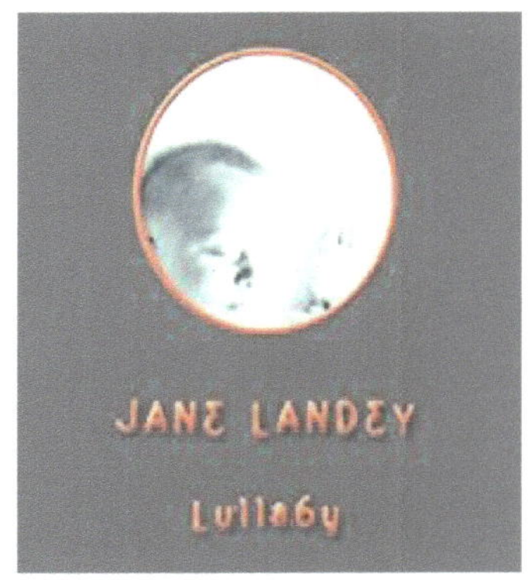

Get your copies at

www.janelandeybookstore.com

the next seeker, and the last is the winner of the round.

THE FIRST STEP IN PLAYING

HIDE AND SEEK

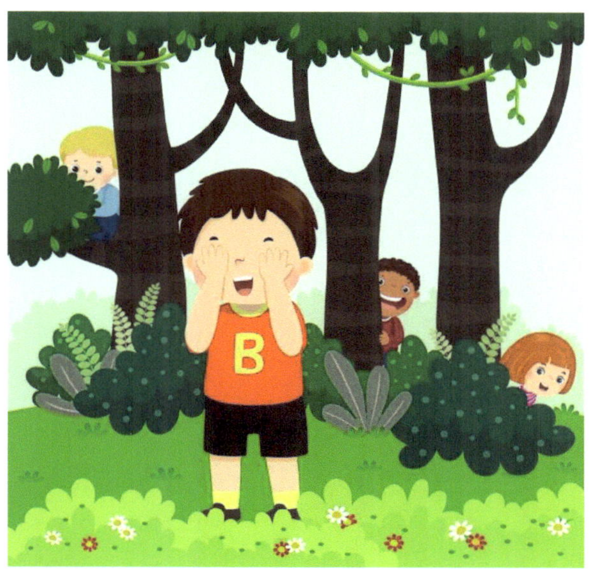

You can play hide-and-seek in real life!

Hide-and-seek is old and popular children's game in which one player closes his or her eyes for a brief period while the other players hide. The seeker then opens his eyes and tries to find the hiders; the first one found is

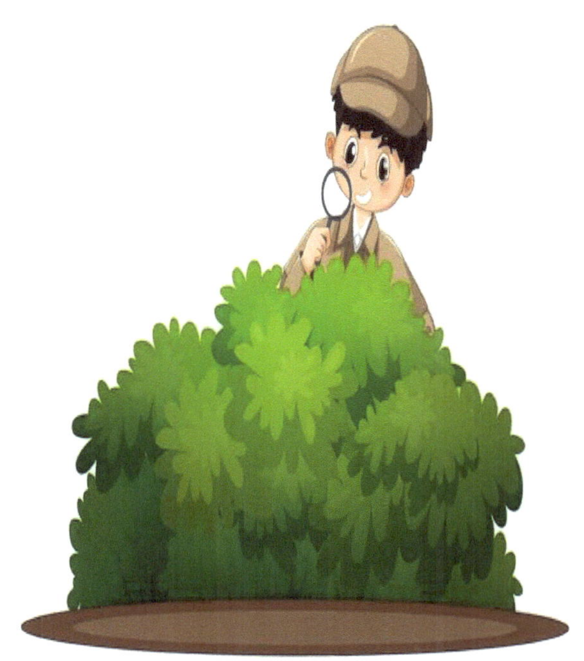

HIDE AND SEEK

Gather at least two players and pick someone to be the seeker. The rest of the players are the hiders. The seeker counts up to 100 while the other players hide. Then, the seeker yells, "Ready or not, here I come!" and starts to search for the hiders.

How to make hide-and-seek more fun

It is more fun to you outside with the group. To play, divide your group into two teams. One team gets time to hide, then the other team starts seeking. The seekers try to capture the hiders and put them in a "jail" of sorts.

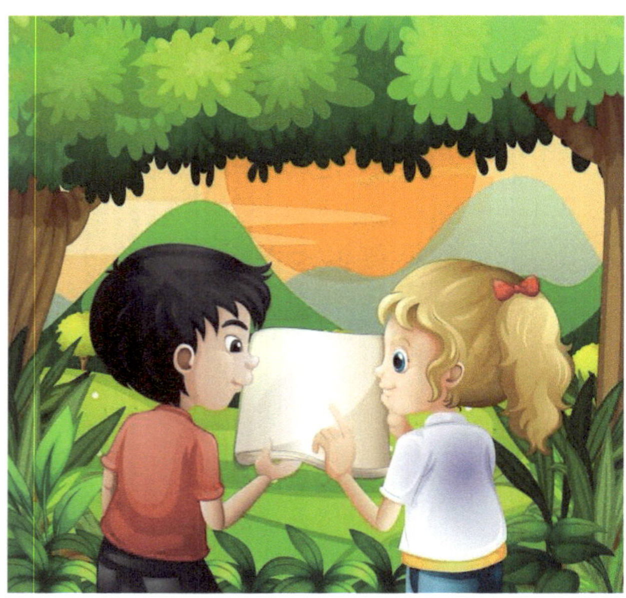

There are different ways to play in teams. Each member of the first team chooses an object which could be a favourite toy or a book. They go and hide so the other team with their eyes closed could search about for the objects.

THE RULES FOR HIDE AND SEEK IN THE DARK

For this version, one person hides, while all the rest of the players try to find them. Once the person in hiding is found, the other seekers try – one by one - to fit into the same hiding place. The game continues till all the players are able to fit into the hiding place and the last seeker finds

How to become a master at Hide and Seek

Look for good hiding spots. Make room for yourself to hide in as many really good spots as you can. Sort out all of the hiding spots that you marked down. Hiding places could be closets, behind shelves, under the table with cover cloth, etc.

PUZZLE

C A R R O T R W P E
P E P P W Q X R U G
C T O M A T O A M G
O V E G C V G D P P
R R T E T O M I K L
N P E P P E R S I A
C A P B A G E H N N
W P O T A T O E S T
C U C U M B E R A Q
W R G D W S A A F I
P O T A F P G T S F

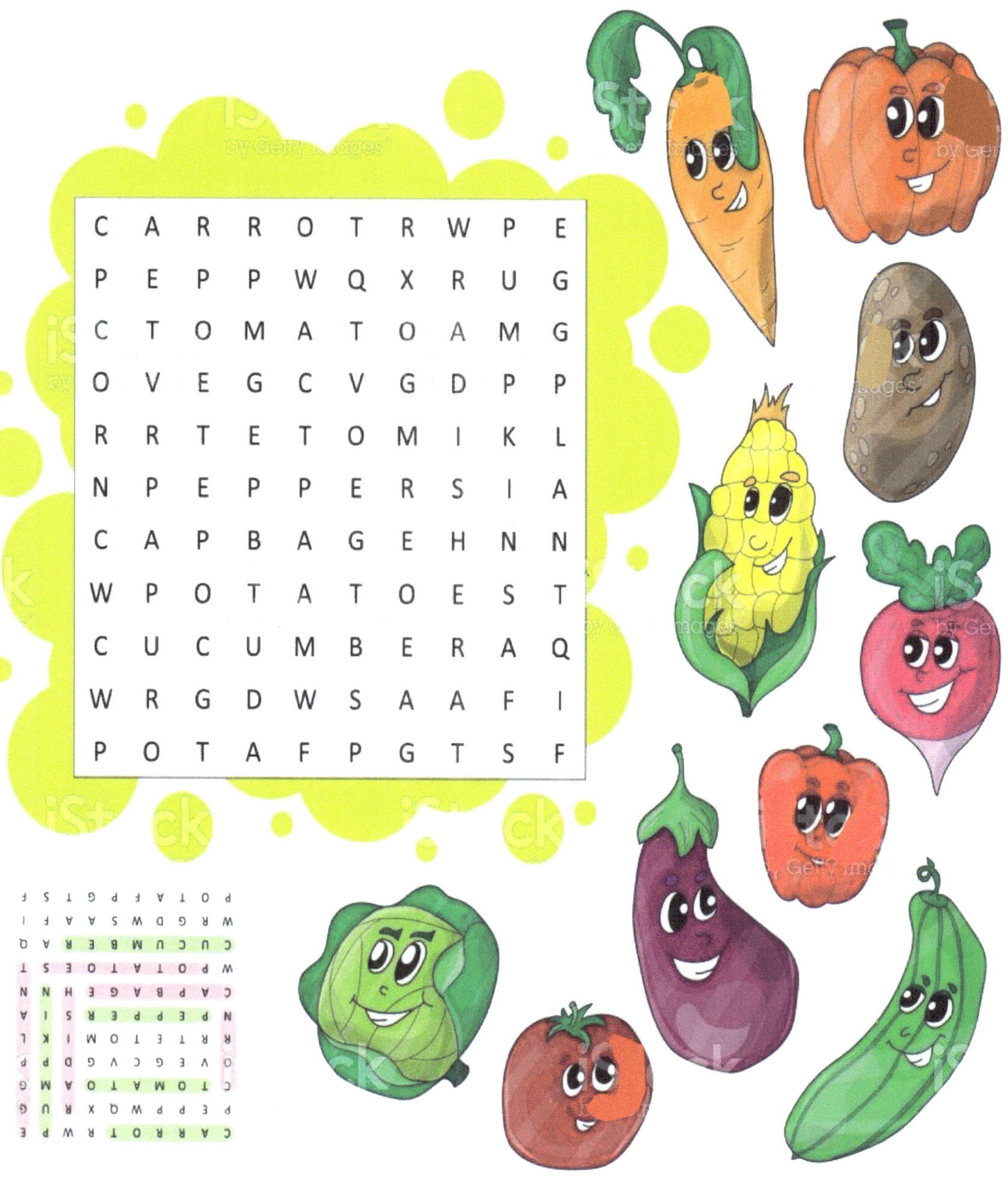

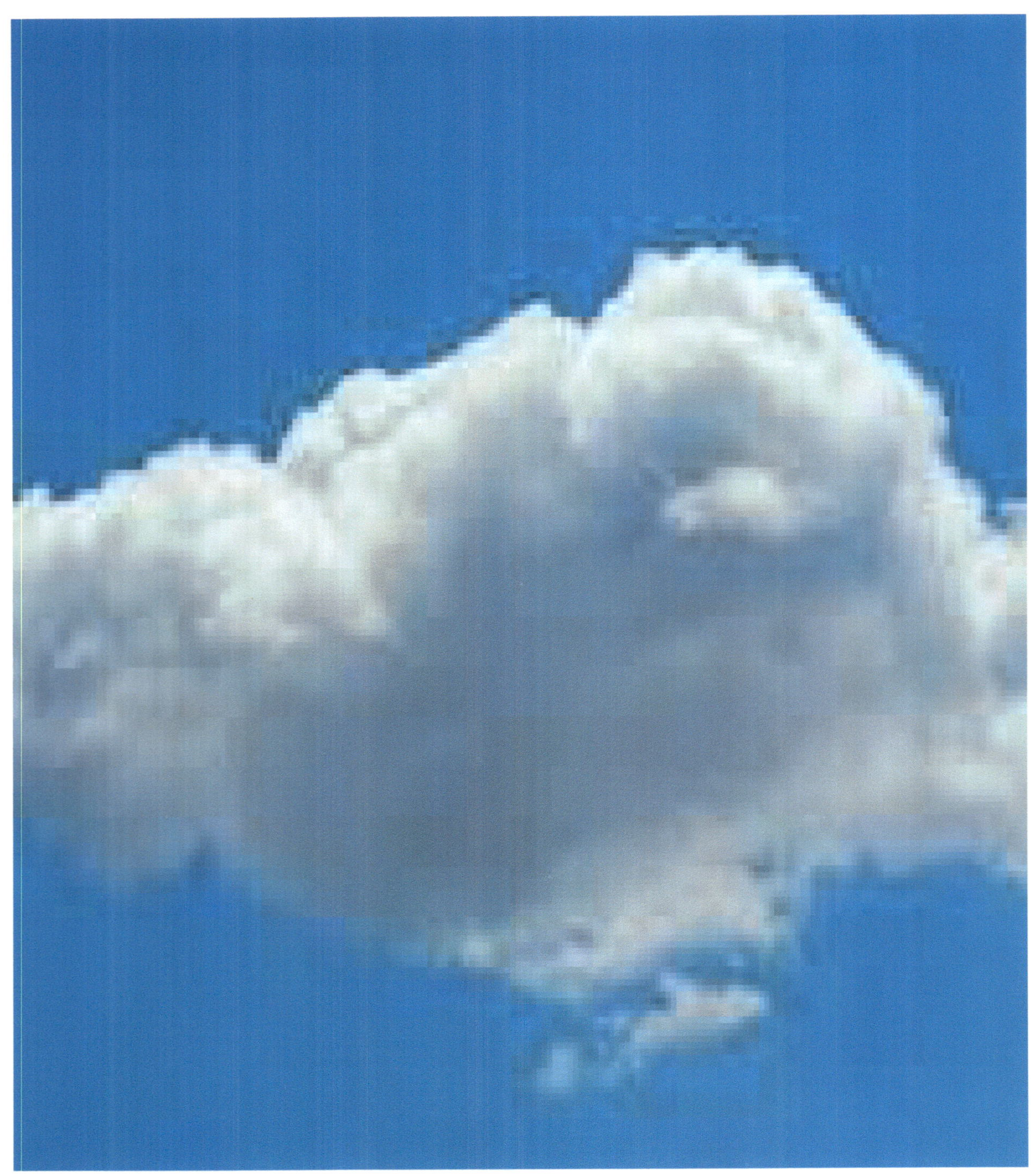

Advice corner by Nikky

Hello, I am here to help you with your problems. Let's get going! What's on your mind? Share it!

Q. Hi Nikky! How long does it take to learn how to play a piano?

A. Beginners can have 4-8 lessons. This will give a beginner knowledge of the keys to play for each tone.

Q. How can I get a good diploma course?

A. You have to know your area of interest. Next step is to search for a good institution that offers it. Finally, enroll and learn hard. Success is at your door!

Q. What do I do to become a good swimmer?

A. Learning how to swim is a bit complex. You must allow someone who is a good swimmer to guide you. You can drown if you learn swimming alone!

Q. Who is the best person to tell your mind?

A. Your father, mother, brother, sister, any close reliable member of your family or close friend can be the best person to confide with your secrete.

Q. I love to eat ice cream. Is it good for my health?

A. It is not advisable to eat ice cream as you eat normal food. That is why it is listed among dessert.

Q. How many hours of sleep is good for me daily?

A.The following is good for each age group daily.

 1 to 2 years, 11 to 14 hours per 24 hours, including naps ; 3 to 5 years, 10 to 13 hours per 24 hours, including naps ; 6 to 12 years, 9 to 12 hours per 24 hours

Most teens need about 8 to 10 hours of sleep each night.

Homework

Arranging the refrigerator

Carpet cleaning

Arranging bookshelf

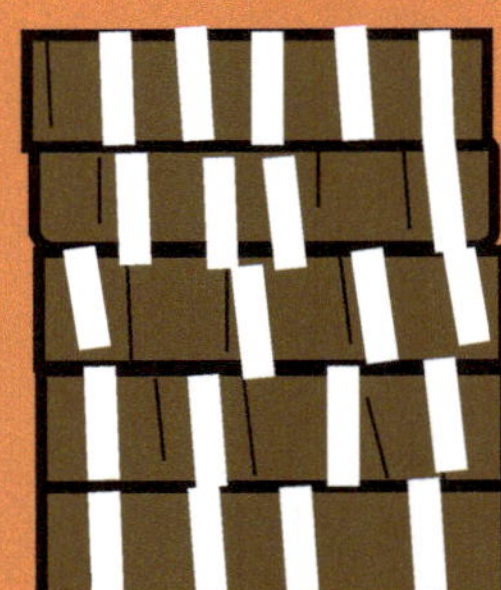

Homework

Yoga

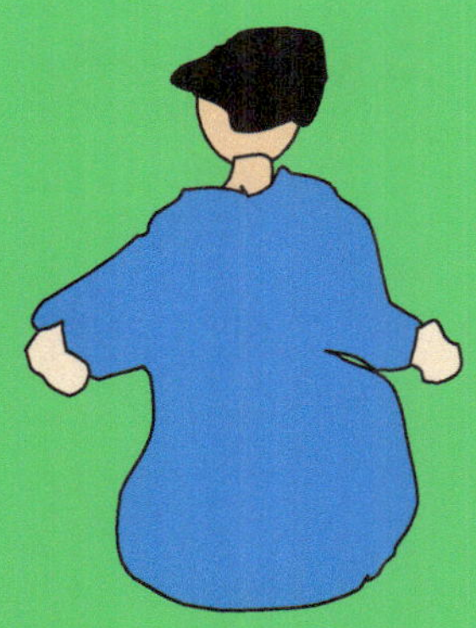

Playing piano

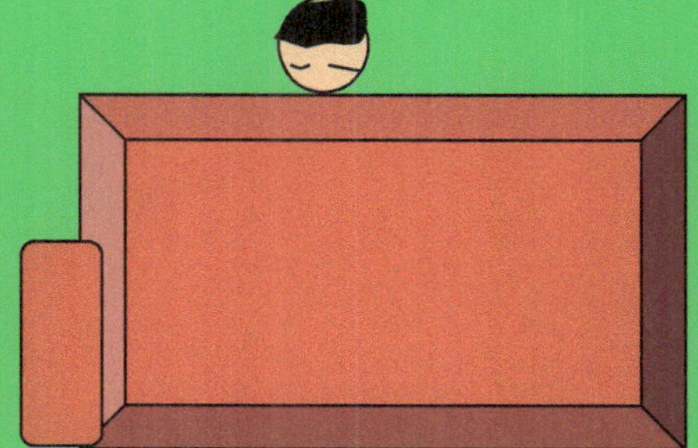

Previously on Young's Delight

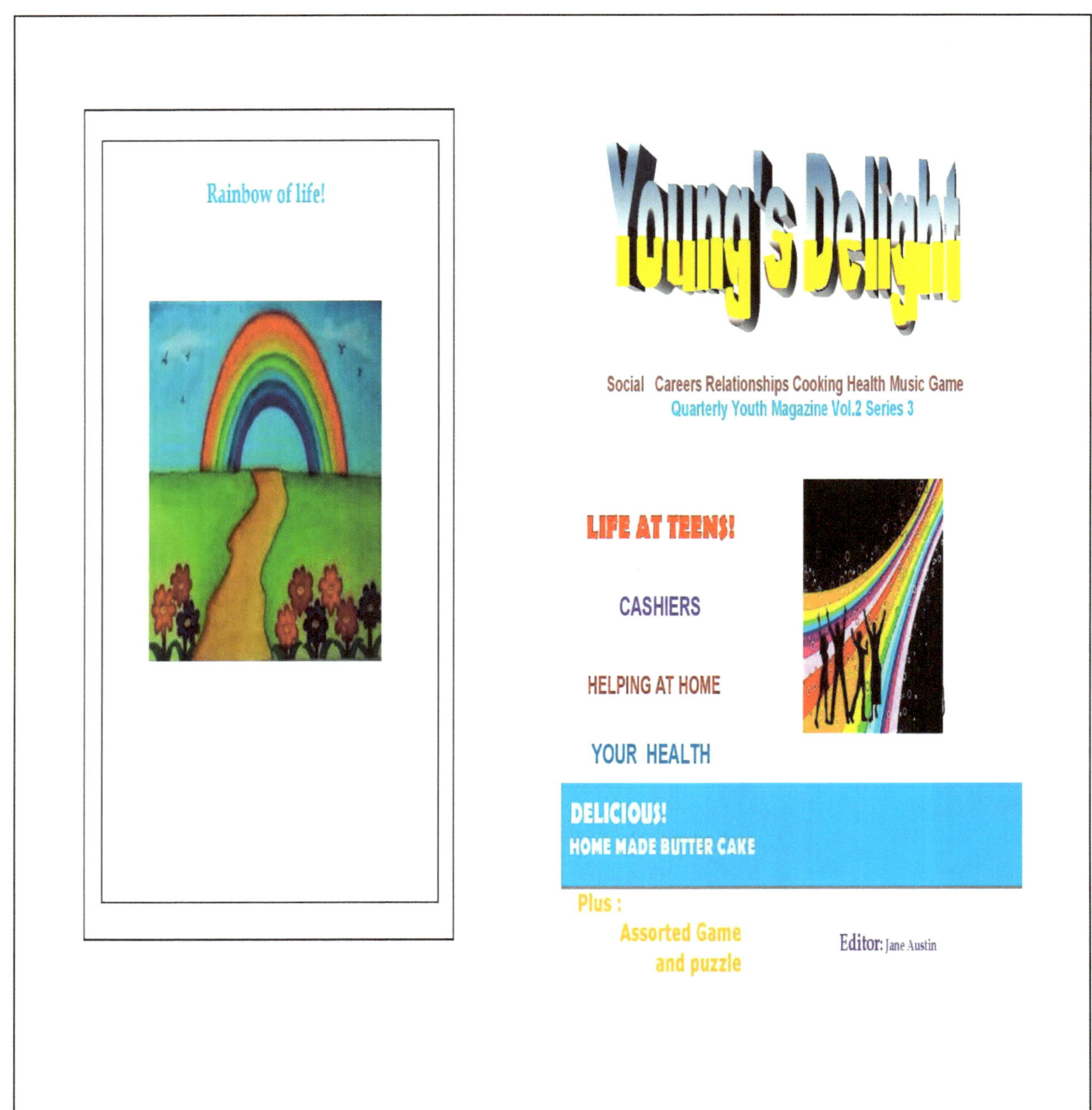

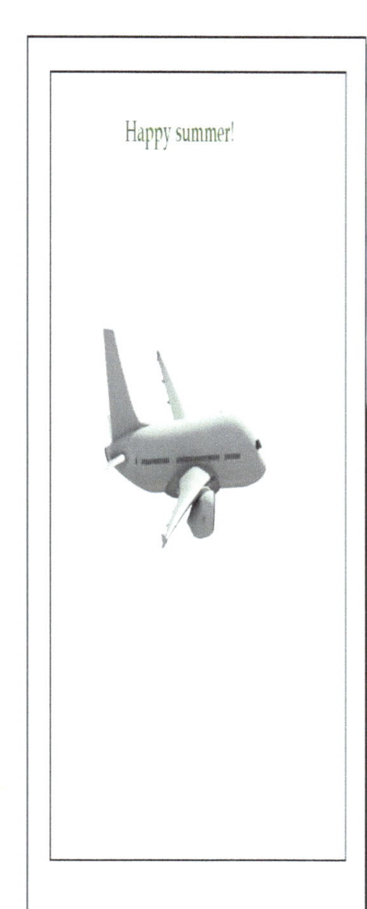

Published by Brims World

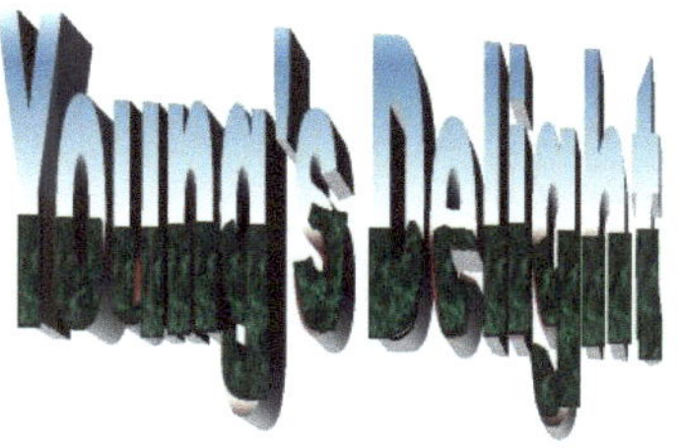

Social   Careers Relationships Cooking Health Music Game
Quarterly Youth Magazine Vol.2 Series 2

ADOLESCENTS!

BECOMING A PILOT

LIFE WITH PARENTS

YOUR HEALTH

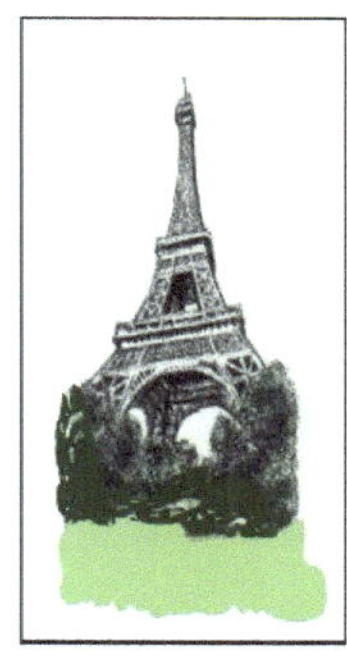

Plus :
Assorted Game
and puzzle

Editor: Jane Austin

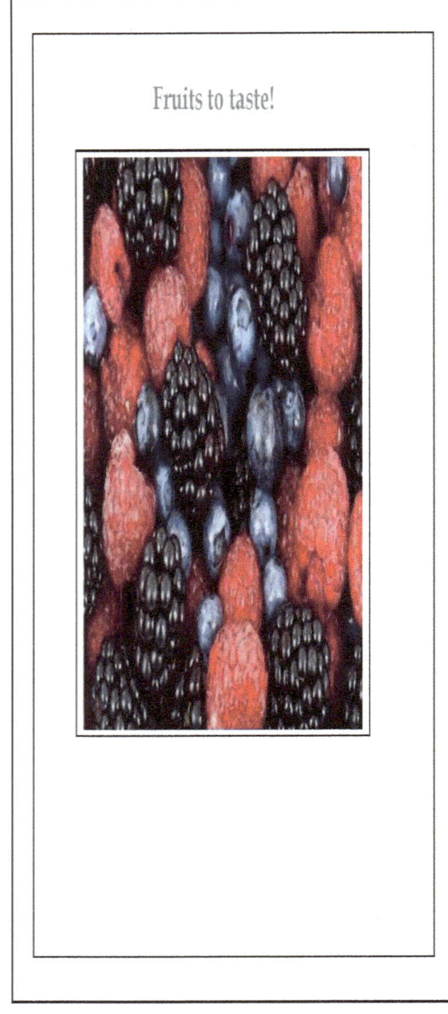

Fruits to taste!

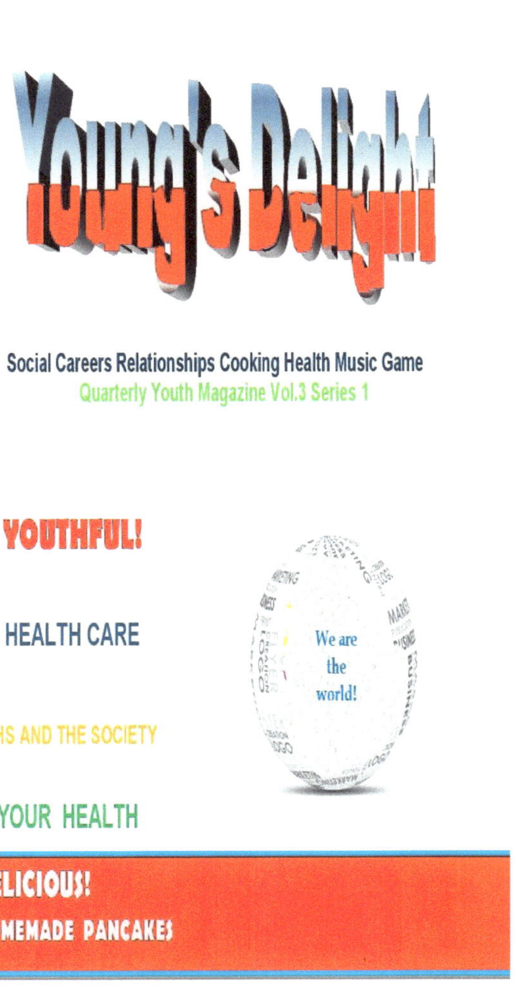

Young's Delight
Social Careers Relationships Cooking Health Music Game
Quarterly Youth Magazine Vol.3 Series 1
YOUTHFUL!
HEALTH CARE
)UTHS AND THE SOCIETY
YOUR HEALTH
We are the world!
DELICIOUS!
HOMEMADE PANCAKES
Plus :
Assorted Game and puzzle
Editor: Jane Austin

Young's Delight

Published by

Brims World L.L.C.

YOUTHS IN THE MAKING

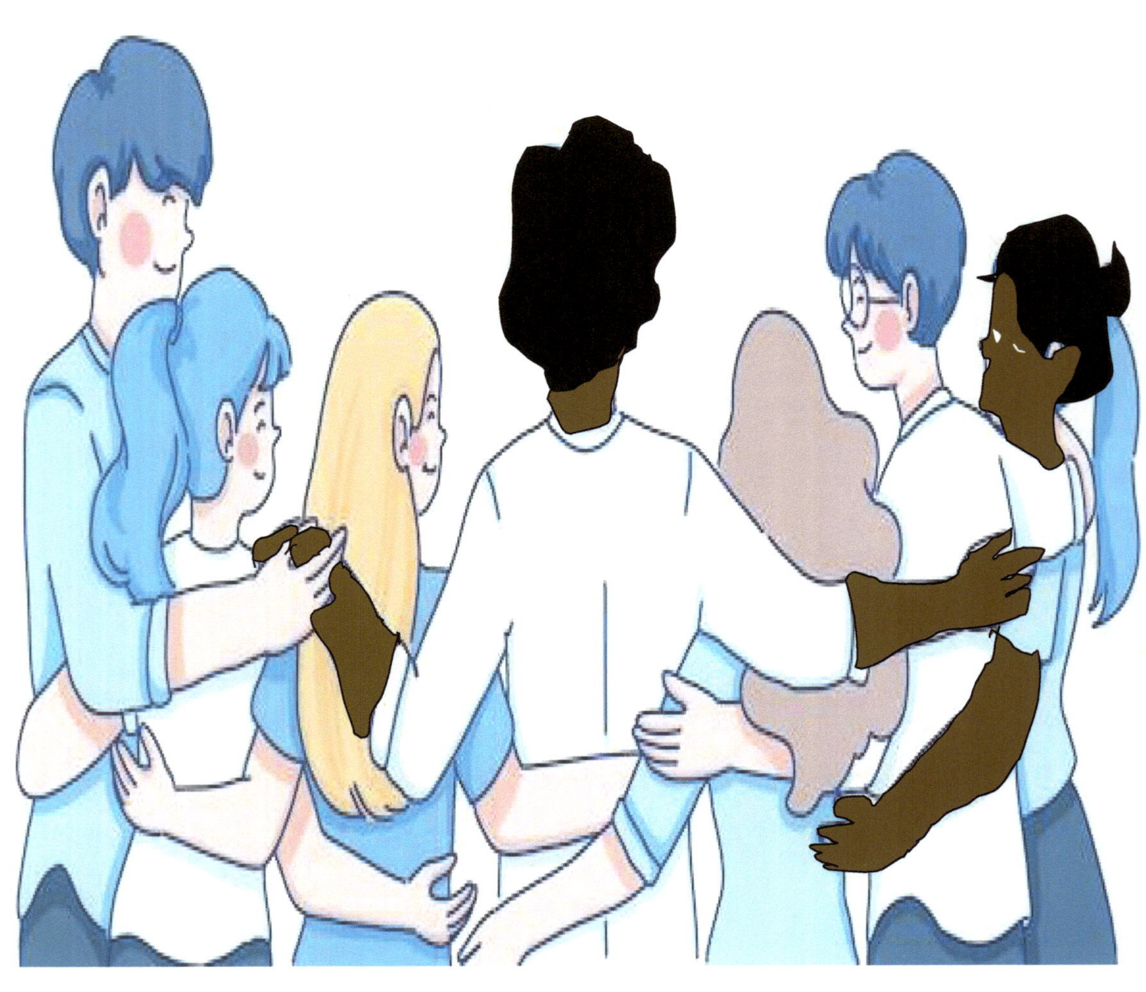

Knowledge.......

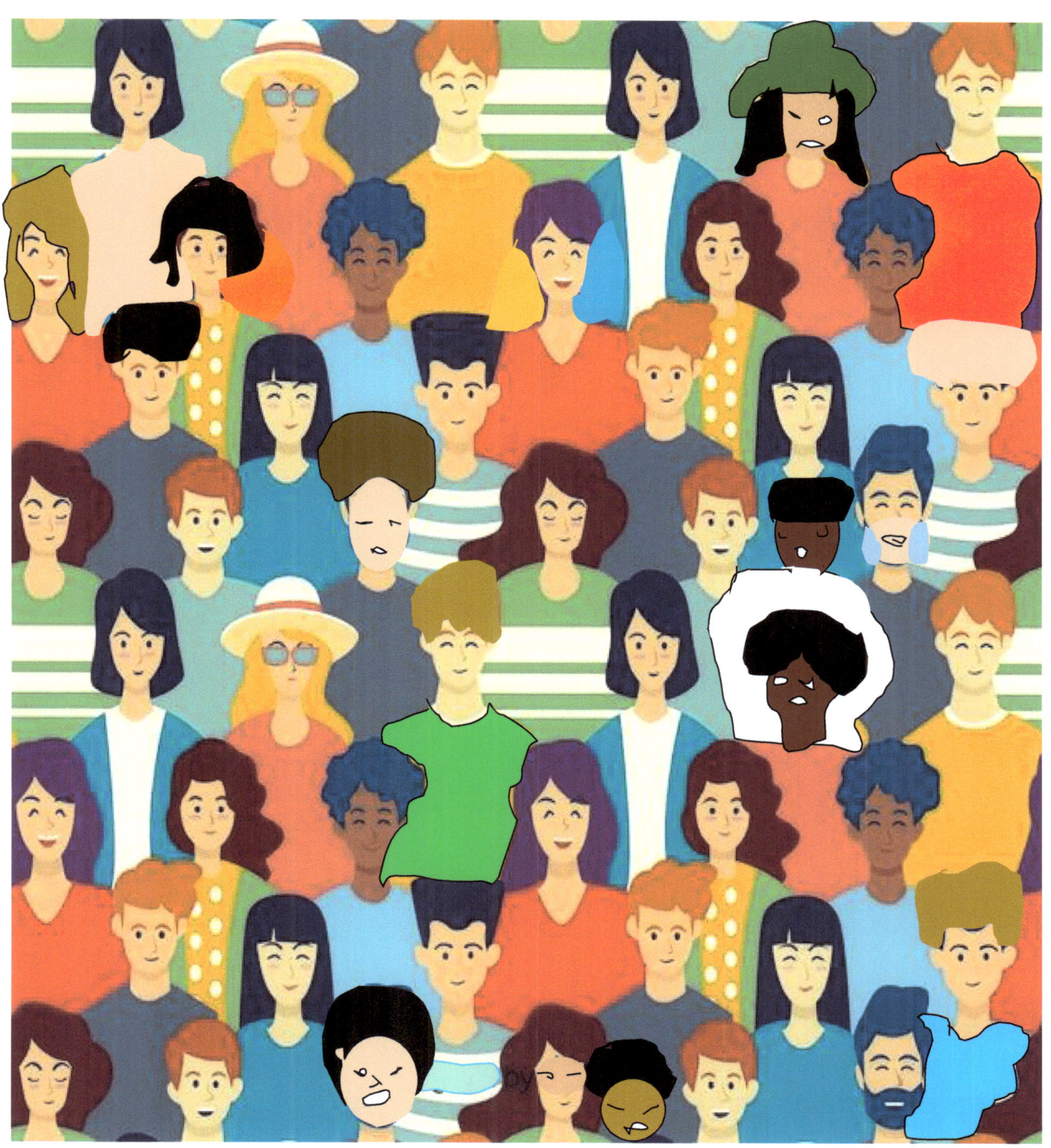

Young's Delight Magazine is published three times in a year. You can subscribe series in unit or yearly bulk.

Send your address and subscription to the following e-mail address:
brimworldincorp1@yahoo.com

Copy the following into your e-mail and send.

Name……………………………………

………………………………………

Address…………………………………

………………………………………

E-mail address……………………………

…………………………..

Unit/Bulk…………………………………

……………………………..

Once we receive your order, we will forward it to your address and inform you through your e-mail address.